CHANGE YOUR BODY, MIND AND LIFE

WELLNESS GUIDE

DANIELA GJURISIC LOJKOVA

BALBOA.
PRESS
A DIVISION OF HAY HOUSE

Balboa Press books may be ordered through booksellers or by contacting:

Balboa Press
A Division of Hay House
1663 Liberty Drive
Bloomington, IN 47403
www.balboapress.com
1 (877) 407-4847

Because of the dynamic nature of the Internet, any web addresses or links contained in this book may have changed since publication and may no longer be valid. The views expressed in this work are solely those of the author and do not necessarily reflect the views of the publisher, and the publisher hereby disclaims any responsibility for them.

The author of this book does not dispense medical advice or prescribe the use of any technique as a form of treatment for physical, emotional, or medical problems without the advice of a physician, either directly or indirectly. The intent of the author is only to offer information of a general nature to help you in your quest for emotional and spiritual well-being. In the event you use any of the information in this book for yourself, which is your constitutional right, the author and the publisher assume no responsibility for your actions.

Any people depicted in stock imagery provided by Thinkstock are models, and such images are being used for illustrative purposes only. Certain stock imagery © Thinkstock.

Print information available on the last page.

ISBN: 978-1-5043-7733-1 (sc)
ISBN: 978-1-5043-7734-8 (hc)
ISBN: 978-1-5043-7735-5 (e)

Library of Congress Control Number: 2017904333

Balboa Press rev. date: 04/07/2017

Contents

Contents

Preface

Let me tell you something that my clients already know, you too can be successful, beautiful, slim, fit, healthy and happy! Yes, you too can change your life into the one you love!

All that I teach, how and where I lead my clients, is based not just on theory that you learn at school or read in a book. My coaching and the program *Training of body and mind,* which I am presenting in this guide, stands on my own experience. I myself and the hundreds of my clients are proof that, if you take the steps I advise, and make a few important changes, you can transform your life into a success story. Your dreams and wishes will come true.

It does not really matter whether you dream of losing weight, becoming fit, earning money, establishing a successful career, or meeting your life partner. I know that when you optimize your nutrition, exercise and thinking, then you tune yourself to success, good health and happiness. It may not be quite clear now how nutrition can be related to your success, but believe me, it is related! Everything is connected to everything else, and success is possible for anyone who is willing to do what it takes to change themselves. You only need to say YES, get up, take the first step and DO your best, and the whole Universe will support you and deliver what you wish for.

Does that sound like an inspirational quote?

Yes! These are inspirational quotes, but they are built on truth.

I want to motivate you!

I want you to tune in!

I want you to take action!

I want you to live the life you love!

I Am Going To Tell You My Story, Why I Became A Wellness Coach

When I was 20 years old, I was overweight and led a bad lifestyle. I suffered from major health problems which doctors couldn't help me with. One day I told myself that enough was enough, and that if the doctors couldn't heal me, then I would change and heal myself. It wasn't easy, but I did it.

I started from scratch to rebuild my lifestyle and seek the best life path. I looked for help in natural medicine, healthy nutrition and exercise. I was also inspired by *You Can Heal Your Life*, a book by Louise Hay, which helped to change my way of thinking.

Honestly, thanks to this experience, I know what it feels like to win! And this feeling is my indicator on the compass. Since that time I have known and felt the right direction forever. I just feel in my bones, in my stomach if I'm on track or if I lost my way.

Step by step I began sharing my experience with others, in order to help them live healthy, happy and successful lives. I had a strong feeling that it was right to share and teach more and more everything I had learned.

I attended various schools and studied everything I could on nutrition therapy, sports, fitness, wellness, massage therapy, psychology, metaphysics, Rciki, etc. I worked with the natural healers, and studied the human body, mind, soul, spirit, herbs, energy healing, as well as exercise and diet. In 2002 I left my job as a real estate broker and became a personal fitness trainer and nutritional therapist and began the first phase of my new profession – teaching people to change their lifestyle, body, mind, and life.

A few years later ...

I attended university and earned a bachelor's degree in sport and fitness and other Wellness and Nutrition specialist diplomas. Based on my knowledge and my own (and my clients') experiences, I developed a program called *Training of body and mind*, which involved 10 steps and taught one of the possible ways to create wellness in body, mind, and spirit. My clientele grew. My clients included celebrities, actors, politicians, businessmen, students, and even entire families. Other experts, such as educators and radio and television journalists, became interested in my program. In 2006, I started teaching at a college and in 2009, I became a co-founder and vice-president of the Alliance of Nutritionists of the Czech Republic. In 2012, I published a book in the Czech language called *Získejte rovnováhu těla, mysli, duše i ducha (Get balance of body, mind, soul and spirit)*. At this time I began to focus mainly on wellness coaching.

I knew and still know that my work in this world is teaching to create wellness in body, mind, and spirit.

NOTE: I AM SURE THAT THE ENTIRE UNIVERSE SUPPORTS OUR EVERY INTENTION AND ALSO SHOWS US THE RIGHT PATH TO FULFILL OUR MISSION IN LIFE.

My story continues ...

Since my teenage years, and even earlier, I dreamt of leaving the Czech Republic, travelling and working abroad. I wanted to share and teach my experience with people all over the world. My call after this dream was so strong and that is why in June 2010 I left my family, my clients, and my great career behind in the Czech Republic and moved to British Columbia, Canada.

I left with minimal knowledge of English. I thought I would spend a couple of years learning English and perhaps work as a housekeeper, but things went differently. After only four months I got a job at a well-known fitness and wellness company in Vancouver, and despite little knowledge of English I quickly became a busy coach.

Now, in 2017, I still live and work in Canada, side by side with a wonderful man and an amazing four-year-old daughter. I run my own wellness and business coaching business, and thanks to the Internet I also work with clients from all over the world. And believe me, I'm not done with my dreams yet. My list is full!

So what about you? What is your story? What is your list of dreams?

I told you my story so that you could understand how powerful the *Training of body and mind* is and how close you are to fulfilling your dreams. Now just say *YES!*, and keep reading.

WARNING: IF YOU ARE EXPERIENCING INJURY OR HAVE A MEDICAL OR HEALTH CONCERN THEN I STRONGLY RECOMMEND YOU CONSULT A PHYSICAL THERAPIST OR OTHER HEALTHCARE PROFESSIONAL BEFORE YOU START MY PROGRAM.

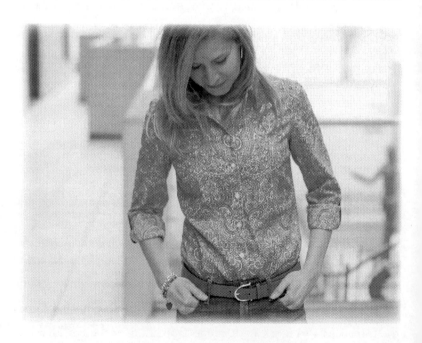

Daniela Gjurisic Lojkova

Introduction

In this book, I will guide you step by step through my program to a successful lifestyle change, which will bring you healthy weight loss, mental and physical fitness and many other benefits beautifying and balancing your whole life. I can promise you that you will make significant progress towards creating wellness in your body, mind, and spirit.

I created this program specifically for you. While my one-on-one coaching is more about you finding your own journey under my guidance, in this program I will show you one particular way in 10 steps. Simple and clearly-stated rules will keep you on track to complete the training successfully and start your new lifestyle.

Various questions will challenge you as you go through the training, and I will give you the answers that are important to you at THAT time. I am sure, all the other answers will come to you at the RIGHT time.

NOTE: FROM MY EXPERIENCE I WOULD RECOMMEND YOU DO NOT BEGIN ANY SIGNIFICANT WORK ON YOUR LIFESTYLE CHANGE UNTIL YOU FINISH READING THIS BOOK AND CREATE A HOLISTIC PICTURE OF THE WHOLE PROGRAM AND THE INDIVIDUAL STEPS. IT IS BENEFICIAL IF YOU

START SLOWLY AND FOLLOW THE ADVICE, BUT REMEMBER, DON'T DO ANYTHING RADICAL UNTIL YOU KNOW ALL 10 STEPS. PLEASE READ THROUGH THE ENTIRE BOOK FIRST, AND THEN GO THROUGH AGAIN AND FOLLOW THE ADVICE STEP BY STEP.

With this guide you will learn:

1. ACHIEVE BALANCE

2. RULES TO GAIN YOUR ORDER AND DISCIPLINE

3. RULES TO MASTER YOUR NUTRITION AND SHOPPING LIST

4. RULES TO MASTER YOUR EXERCISE AND FITNESS SCHEDULE

5. RULES TO MASTER YOUR THOUGHTS

6. TO CALCULATE YOUR OPTIMUM BODY WEIGHT

7. TO DO BODY MEASUREMENTS

8. TO SET THE DEADLINE BY WHICH YOU WILL LOSE WEIGHT

9. TO FACE FEAR

10. TO DO YOUR VERY BEST

Before We Begin, I Must Warn You

This program opens the door to a new world! It is targeted primarily at the body and mind but also touches the spirit, because everything is connected to everything else!

With this program you will begin major changes in your life. You will speed up your metabolism, begin to reduce body fat, change body composition, heal, restore and rebalance yourself. You will increase your energy and fitness level, as well as your creativity and intuition. Stress, joint pains, abdominal pain, back pain, allergies, migraine, high cholesterol, and similar inconveniences will gradually migrate or completely disappear. You will again feel young physically as well as mentally. You will become an active, positive, satisfied, fit and balanced person. That's beautiful! Yes, that's what you want.

However, get ready for the fact that you will change not only the body and mind but also something from your surroundings to which you have been accustomed. Which is not bad, it's just a process of transformation and healing on all levels. For example, you may lose some of your relationships, but for sure you will get new ones that will suit you better. It's like when you clean your house and giving away things no longer needed. Well, you may lose some of your friends, and get a new awesome one who will enjoy your new lifestyle. You may change your occupation, or residence, to get better like those you have been dreaming about. You maybe buy a pet, even if you never even thought about it. Many things can happen. But surely, you will change your wardrobe.

And of course, prepare yourself to live a very long and active life. Instead of slippers and a rocking chair, you'll be buying sneakers and a bike! Are you ready for all that? Are you ready that in your 50s, 60s, 70s, and maybe even your 80s, you will ski, run marathons, play tennis, travel, and go out on a date?

Do you want that?

Yes, of course you do! That's why you're here! So let's get started!

Clarifying The "Aging Process"

Have you ever noticed that whatever you do, whether you're surfing the Internet, reading a magazine, newspaper or book, watching the television, listening to the radio, whether you are at work, driving in your car, riding the bus, or just walking down the street you always see and hear the words: obesity, overweight, cardiovascular disease, high blood pressure, high cholesterol, diabetes, allergies, indigestion, poor immunity, joint pain, back pain, arthritis, osteoporosis, premenstrual syndrome, menopause, stroke, heart attack, tiredness, and stress? Of course you have!

Well, some doctors argue that the cause of these problems is simply the aging process of your body, but studies, research and results have shown that these problems may never appear at all if we maintain a healthy lifestyle and pay attention to wellness in body, mind, and spirit. And I for one completely agree with that.

So, here we are at the beginning of your new, beautiful, fit, healthy and happy life.

Let's take the first step.

Training Of Body And Mind In 10 Steps

Training of Body and Mind is built on three essential pillars:

1. Optimized and balanced NUTRITION

2. Optimized and balanced EXERCISE

3. Optimized and balanced THOUGHTS

REMEMBER: EVERY TIME YOU ARE GOING TO FULFILL A NEW GOAL, IMAGINE THAT JUST THIS GOAL IS SITTING ON THE LAST STEP OF THE STAIRS. GO UP THE STAIRS AND LEARN WHAT YOU NEED TO LEARN ON THE FIRST STEP, THEN GO UP THE NEXT STEP, LEARN, AND THE NEXT, LEARN, AND THE NEXT, UNTIL YOU REACH THE LAST ONE. IT'S A GAME! PLAY WITH IT LIKE A LITTLE KID AND YOU WILL REACH WHATEVER YOU DECIDE. JUST SAY YES AND DO YOUR VERY BEST. THROW AWAY ALL THE *SHOULD*, AND GO FOR IT. IF YOU DO A GOOD THING, THEN THE WHOLE UNIVERSE WILL SUPPORT YOU AND HELP YOU.

Take a deep breath, we're going to take the first step!

Step 1

The Balance

If you take away only one thing from this book, please let it be the word BALANCE.

Repeat after me: Balance, balance, balance

And once more: Balance

Balance is essential for the whole life as well as to THE WHOLE being! Think about it. If you can't maintain balance, you fall down. Without balance you can't even take one step. When your muscles are not balanced, you feel pain. Without balance of internal and external environment the human body is sick or dies. Balance applies to everything – money, health, thinking, relationships, jobs, diet, exercise, healthy weight, everything.

REMEMBER: KEEP THE BALANCE OF BODY, MIND, SOUL AND SPIRIT AND YOU WILL SEE HOW MIRACLES CAN HAPPEN AND HOW YOUR LIFE CAN SMOOTHLY CHANGE FOR THE BETTER. WHAT YOU GIVE OUT COMES BACK TO YOU. YOU GET AS MUCH AS YOU GIVE.

NOTE: THINK ABOUT BALANCE WHEN YOU READ THIS BOOK, WHEN YOU WORK OUT, WHEN YOU COOK, EAT, WORK, THINK, SLEEP OR PLAY WITH CHILDREN.

Notes:

_____

_____

_____

_____

_____

_____

_____

_____

_____

_____

_____

_____

_____

Step 2

The Personal Daily Journal

Trust me when I say that a journal plays an important role in the whole process of a lifestyle change and weight loss.

An expert could say that keeping a journal is old-fashioned but who cares? I know it works very well so why not take advantage of it?

A journal helps in setting and maintaining rules, order, discipline, motivation and attention. It also helps you remember goals and rules, keep track of what you eat, drink, exercise, think and clearly see an improvement in your body weight and measurement. A journal works as a good friend who gives you the true feedback and shows your progress.

What kind of journal you choose is completely up to you. Clarity is important. You'll use your journal several times a day and carry it with you. I suggest that you choose a reasonable size journal with a moderate number of pages.

The rules to master your journal:

1. **Track F-E-T-E-G – every day:**

   * Food and drinks – What, when, and how much you eat and drink during the day.

   * Exercise – What type of movement, and how much time you exercise during the day.

   * Thoughts – What you think, such as new ideas or questions.

   * Experience – One enjoyable experience every day. Ask yourself: What went great today?

   * Goals – Make a list of 2 new goals you want to accomplish for the next day. At first, they should relate to this program. Every night before bedtime, check them off if you complete them.

2. **Track Body Weight – every Monday:**

   * Weight and record your weight every Monday morning before breakfast. You will receive further instructions in Step 6.

3. Track Body Measurement – every second Monday:

* When you enter into Step 7, than begin to Measure and record your body measurement every second Monday. You will receive further instructions in Step 7.

This step was not so bad, right? So go out and buy a nice journal, and then follow me on the next step.

Notes:

Step 3

Optimized And Balanced Nutrition

You should understand that your metabolism is exactly like fire. Keeping your metabolism burning is like keeping a good fire burning. If you want fire in the fireplace, you must stoke the fire with the right wood. If you want fire in the body, you must use the right food.

The rules to master your food:

1. Basic rules for healthy eating:

    *   Keep your **caloric intake** between 1500-2000 Kcal per day if you are a woman, and 2000-2500 Kcal per day if you are a man.

    *   **Eat 3-5 portions** per day. Bigger breakfast, smaller lunch and small dinner + 1 small snack throughout the day.

    *   Eat the **right amount** of healthy balanced food depending on how active you are.

    *   Keep the **right value** of carbohydrates, protein, fat, fibre, vitamins and minerals.

* Keep the **right percentage ratio** of carbohydrates, proteins and fats, per

DAY:

50% carbs of daily energy intake (no more than 10% of sugar)

25% protein of daily energy intake and between 0.7 and 1 gram of protein per kg of body weight. Warning: High protein diet can increase health risks!

25% fat of daily energy intake (80% unsaturated fat, 20% saturated fat).

MEAL:

Breakfast: High carbs + medium protein + small amount of fat intake.

Lunch: Medium carbs + medium protein + small amount of fat intake.

Dinner: Low carbs + medium protein + small amount of fat intake.

EXERCISE - Before and after sport/exercise:

90 min before workout: Complex carbs; small amount of protein; small amount of fat; really small amount of fibre.

90 min after workout: Medium carbs; medium protein; small amount of fat intake.

* Keep a **break of 2-4 hours** between each meal (snack).

* **Avoid** eating **carbs after 2pm.**

* Finish **dinner at 6**-7pm.

* Avoid eating at **night** (after 7pm).

* **Never** try to **starve yourself.**

* **Plan your meals** and snacks in advance.

* Do **not eat the same** food every day.

* Eat **colourfully.**

* Eat **fresh** food every day.

* Eat **RAW or gently cooked** food.

* Choose **NATURAL / ORGANIC** food as much as possible.

* Reduce intake of **gluten** and **acid-forming** foods.

* Choose the right food for maintaining **proper pH levels** in the body, as much as possible.

* Stay **away from junk**, processed and **GMO** food, with preservatives and chemicals.

* Follow the general principles of food **hygiene.**

* Read **food labels.**

* **Listen** to your body.

* Choose 1 day a week when you can eat one regular portion of **your favourite meal** or sweet.

* Use a daily food **journal** to keep track of your food.

2. **Say YES to this food:**

Your diet should include the following range of foods.

* HEALTHY CARBS

    Whole grains, beans, fruit and vegetables. Potatoes, legumes, cereals, peas, lentils, beans, oats, millet. Choose whole grain varieties whenever possible – bread, brown rice, millet, quinoa, barley, fruits and vegetables.

    + FRUITS AND VEGETABLES

        There are many fruit and vegetables with lots of health benefits. Eat fresh and organic as much as possible. I recommend you eat seasonal fruit and vegetables grown in your region or country, for which your body is tuned. Reduce the amount of tropical fruit you consume (especially in the winter) unless you actually live in a tropical climate.

* HEALTHY FATS

Fats from plants, seeds, and fish help reduce bad cholesterol (LDL) in your blood, and help develop and maintain your body's cells.

+ **Monounsaturated fatty acids** – From many plants, nuts and seeds, such as olives, canola, peanuts, sunflowers, sesame, avocados, almonds, hazelnuts, pecans, pumpkin, sesame.

+ **Polyunsaturated fatty acids** – Omega-3 and Omega-6 – fatty fish, such as salmon, herring, mackerel, anchovies, sardines, and unheated sunflower oil, flaxseed oil, soybean oil, corn oil, walnut oil. Choose cold pressed varieties whenever possible.

* HEALTHY PROTEIN

Fish, turkey, beans, nuts, seeds, and eggs. The key is variety. Eat at least two portions of fish, seafood, or seaweed every week. Eat at least one portion of lean and skinless chicken or turkey every week. Choose only fermented milk products, such as cottage cheese and plain yogurt, fat-free or low-fat varieties whenever possible.

＊ SPICES AND HERBS

There are many spices and herbs with numerous health benefits. Use fresh and organic as much as possible. Among my favourites are cinnamon, ginger root, parsley, sage, rosemary, calendula officinalis, basil, pepper, caraway seeds, clove, and garlic.

＊ WATER

Helps flush your body of waste products and toxins and burn up your metabolism. Drink six to eight glasses of water per day. When it is a hot day, drink more. Drink warm rather than cold water.

Start your day with a glass of warm fresh lemon-water to balance your pH levels, clean your body, boosts your immune system, stimulate bowel movements, and get many other important benefits.

＊ HIGH IN POTASSIUM & LOW IN SODIUM DIET

Avocado, apricot, banana, and a variety of green vegetables, such as kale, spinach, and lettuce. Potassium is naturally present in most fruits and vegetables. Sodium (salt) is naturally present in all foods, even fruit and vegetables. But salt is also added into a lot of food!

* ORGANIC

Choose organic as much as possible.

REMEMBER: DO NOT STOP EATING, JUST CHANGE THE WAY YOU EAT. DO NOT GO ON A STRONG DIET, JUST DO STOP EATING THE WRONG FOOD.

3. Say NO to this food:

The following should be reduced or eliminated from your diet.

* BAD CARBS

Cut them down as much as possible.

- **Refined sugar** – Lower the consumption of this as much as possible.

- **White flour and gluten** - You need to significantly reduce white flour and intake of gluten as much as possible.

NOTE: THE COLOUR OF THIS TYPE OF CARBS IS <u>WHITE</u>.

* BAD FATS

Cut them down as much as possible.

- **Saturated fats** – Raises your bad (LDL) cholesterol and lowers your good (HDL) cholesterol. Increases your risk of heart disease, stroke, overweight, obesity and type 2 diabetes. Comes from animal sources (meat – beef, lamb, pork, poultry with skin), whole milk dairy products (butter, lard, milk, cheese, cream, creamy yogurts, and other dairy products made from 2 or more percent fat milk). Some oils from plants contain primarily saturated fats, but do not contain cholesterol (palm oil, palm kernel oil and coconut oil).

- **Trans fats** (or trans-unsaturated fatty acids) – Type of unsaturated fats that are uncommon in nature and have been implicated in serious health problems. Comes from processed food made of hydrogenated vegetable oil, fried food, baked goods (usually packaged), cakes, pie crusts, biscuits, frozen pizza, cookies, crackers, candies, margarines.

NOTE: WHEN THIS TYPE OF FAT IS COOLED, ITS COLOUR IS <u>WHITE</u>.

* SALT, PRESERVATIVES AND CHEMICALS

- Canned food, sausage, candy, roasted nuts and seeds. Warning: 1g of sodium is equivalent to

2.5g of salt. Salt is essential for our good health, however, no more than 5g a day for adults is needed. High sodium and low potassium intakes can increase health risks including high blood pressure, cardiovascular disease, and stroke.

* FRIED FOOD

* BURNED FOOD

* PRESERVED FOOD

* PROCESSED FOOD

* ROTTEN FOOD

* GMO FOOD

* ACID-FORMING FOOD

* ALCOHOL

* BLACK COFFEE AND TEA (CAFFEINE)

* TOBACCO

* DRUGS

WARNING: READ FOOD LABELS. FOOD OR INGREDIENTS OF *NO* GROUP MAY BE ADDED IN FOOD AND DRINKS OF *YES* GROUP.

REMEMBER: WHENEVER YOU SEE WHITE-COLOURED FOOD, THINK TWICE. ASK YOURSELF IN WHICH FOOD GROUP IT BELONGS. I AM NOT SAYING THAT ALL WHITE FOOD IS BAD.

THE BALANCE IS THE KEY TO WEIGHT MANAGEMENT.

* THAT MEANS IF YOU WANT TO LOSE WEIGHT, YOU NEED TO REDUCE ENERGY INTAKE (LESS FOOD) AND INCREASE ENERGY EXPENDITURE (MORE EXERCISE).

* YOU HAVE TO MAKE A LIFESTYLE CHANGE = YOU HAVE TO CHANGE YOUR WAY OF THINKING, STOP EATING THE WRONG FOOD, AND DO REGULAR EXERCISE.

Well done!

HOMEWORK:

Now take a highlighter, please, and select five rules that attract you most and that you will apply to your life from this moment on. Also, make two copies of *the rules to master your food* and hang one on the fridge and place the other on the nightstand.

Then, every second Monday take a highlighter and select one more rule. Write down this regular homework into your journal and calendar too!

Done? Great.

Master your shopping list:

Never write a shopping list when you're hungry. Likewise, never shop for food when you're hungry!

Please read this step once again and then think of the possibilities of your new diet and about specific foods that you will need to buy. Ask family members for their ideas and suggestions. They might join you and follow a healthy diet with you. Make a shopping list. Bear in mind that you can buy organic products online.

Already done? Then you're on the right track!

NOTE: AT THE END OF THIS BOOK, IN THE CATEGORY OF BONUSES, YOU WILL FIND MEAL TIPS AND AN EXAMPLE OF A WEEKLY MENU PLANNER TO HELP YOU WITH COMPLETING YOUR FINAL SHOPPING LIST.

Let's jump to the next step.

Notes:

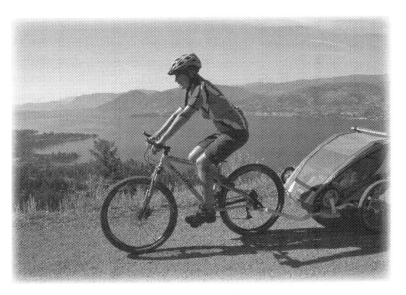

Daniela Gjurisic Lojkova

Step 4

Optimized And Balanced Exercise

The right movement will increase your metabolism and speed up the rate at which you burn calories and fat. Moreover, it will tone your body and keep you fit.

The rules to master your muscles:

1. Strength (resistance) training

This type of movement is essential for building healthy muscles and strong bones.

* Do 45-60 minutes, 3-4 times a week.

* Work out at a variety of intensity levels to tap into different energy systems.

* Alternate medium and high levels. To achieve this level you have to train, so start with a low intensity and gradually increase.

* Each muscle group should be worked on two or more days each week. It's fine if you begin on one day a

week, and as you gradually increase your fitness level you raise the number to two or more.

* Alternate strength, plyometric and body weight exercises.

* If you are a beginner, then start with strength training in the gym and after a few workouts gradually add plyometric and core exercises.

* Hire a personal trainer for at least for the first month (12 sessions) of your new exercise plan. The trainer will teach you suitable exercises and a proper technique.

REMEMBER: STEP BY STEP IS THE RIGHT WAY.

2. Aerobic exercise in moderate heart rate zone (60 to 70 percent of HRmax)

This type of movement is important, or rather necessary in maintaining a strong and healthy cardiovascular system, to speeds up metabolism, burns fat, ensures healthy weight loss and the regeneration and renewal of cells and tissues and to keep you young.

Do 45-60 minutes without <u>any</u> break, 4-5 times a week, in heart zone 60-70% of HRmax. I'd love to see you doing intervals 2-3 times a week, where you alternate high and low resistance: 6-minute warm up + 1-minute higher resistance and 70-75% HR max + 2-minute lower resistance and 55-60%

HRmax, repeat this scheme, last six minutes calm down to lower resistance and HR. Plus training twice a week with constant resistance.

I recommend you alternate between the following: elliptical trainer, bike ride, power walk and slow run.

HOMEWORK:

Calculate your heart rate:

Use the formula:

$HRmax = 220$ - *age in years* $=$

HR *(60%)* $= HRmax \times 0.60 =$

HR *(70%)* $= HRmax \times 0.70 =$

3. Stretching and relaxation

The following is particularly necessary to ensure a speedy recovery, excellent flexibility, and healthy joints and muscles.

* Stretch your muscles before and after each workout for 10-15 min.

* Stretch your muscles every day for at least 15-20 min.

* Take a relaxing massage or energy healing (for example Reiki) at least every second week.

* Sleep 8 hours per day.

I recommend you practice the slow version of the classic yoga, which is an ideal way to relax, stretch and meditate.

NOTE: AT THE END OF THE BOOK, IN THE CATEGORY OF BONUSES, YOU CAN FIND EXAMPLES OF THE WORKOUTS.

Easy, right? You have just mastered the second pillar of *Training of body and mind*! Most of my clients are surprised about the need for aerobic exercise and strength training at the same time. Many of them also do not know the proper rules of aerobic exercise. What about you?

Now, guess what …

HOMEWORK:

Please, take a highlighter, and choose one rule that attracts you most (Resistance training or Aerobic exercise or Stretching and relaxation) that you will apply to your life from this moment on. Also, make two copies of *the rules to master your muscles* and hang one on the fridge and place the other on the nightstand.

Then, every second Monday take a highlighter and select another rule. Write down this regular homework into your journal and calendar too!

Done? Great.

Now before we move forward I have an important message for you, and that is ...

Whatever I have ever said, I am now saying that you need to train in the gym!

If we worked together one-on-one, then I would say you can do your workouts at home, because as a trainer I would make sure how, when, and what you exercise. But we do not have that possibility. So you have to go to the gym! Remember, you have a goal! So, do the best you can! Light walking, burning calories during ironing, or exercising at home on the carpet between cooking dinner, is not enough! You have to go to a place where they have sports equipment, free weights, machines, elastic ropes, balloons and bicycles. You need to sweat, you need to lift weights and really feel your muscles burn! You have to see others train. You have to see young people and seniors, men and women, what they do and how they do it. All this will give you motivation, inspiration, and, most importantly, no one (no husbands, kids, friends, or bosses) will disturb you there!

Even better if you can hire a personal trainer ...

At least for the first month (12 sessions) of your new exercise plan. He/she will teach you how and what to train, and be there to help and support you. The first month of diet and exercise is the most important. You will be in new surroundings, you will hurt your muscles, you will learn new things, you will eat different food, and you will have a new time schedule. You will need courage, faith, discipline and support, and a personal trainer can help you with this. Paying for lessons and having a trainer waiting for you will help keep you focused and force you to train. If you pass the first month, you will be that much closer to victory.

HOMEWORK:

Now, please turn on your computer and search the Internet for the nearest gym in your area. Choose your favourite one and make an appointment for a free fitness orientation.

Done? Beautiful! You rock!

Master your fitness schedule:

Don't forget that your husband or wife, your kids, and probably even your dog are going to participate in your new schedule. So you need to create a plan that works for everyone involved.

Have you thought about your new time schedule? Which days are you going to work out, do aerobic exercise, or meditate?

You can use the table below to write out your plan. Take a pen and paper and find a quiet and undisturbed place. Think of various possibilities. Light a candle and write down everything that comes to mind. After that, circle your 10 best ideas. Make sure to consult with your family. I like the words *for the good of all involved* very much, because it gives free will to all.

Here's an idea of what your new beginner's fitness schedule might look like:

	Aerobic	Workout	Relax
Monday	55 min speed walk		
Tuesday			30 min meditation
Wednesday	50 min elliptical in the gym	Gym – upper body	
Thursday			
Friday	50 min elliptical in the gym	Gym – lower body	
Saturday	60 min speed walk		
Sunday		Core training at home	

Your own fitness schedule:

	Aerobic	Workout	Relax
Monday			
Tuesday			
Wednesday			
Thursday			
Friday			
Saturday			
Sunday			

Done? Let me see.

I like your new schedule very much!

Now you are ready to move on the next step.

Notes:

Step 5

Optimized And Balanced Thoughts

Positive thoughts are an extremely powerful tool!

It is essential that you understand the power of POSITIVE THINKING. After years of practice, I have learned that this part is the most important thing in life. Not food or exercise, but the way of thinking and speaking. If you want to be happy, successful and loved, then this is your number one! Trust me!

If you haven't started to practice it yet, then you have to start RIGHT NOW, because your wonderful life comes from it.

I believe that we work much like a computer and can be programmed like a computer too. A computer's behaviour depends on the program you load into it and so it is with us, human beings. I am deeply convinced that if you program yourself to love and positive direction, then everything in your body and life will work in a positive direction as well.

The level of body, mind and spirit interact. Each cell is affected by each piece of food, each movement, each emotion, and also by each thought. Absolutely everything around us and within us is constantly affecting us, whether you can feel it or not.

You can be "*infected*" by the situation, person, group of people, the environment, books, television, radio, music, mood, colour, words, pictures, and others; and each time, it can be either positive or negative. Positive is perfectly fine, enjoy that to the fullest. But avoid and protect yourself from negative.

The rules to master your thoughts:

1. **Stop complaining**

   * About yourself! About how you look and feel about your work and life.

   * About how difficult it is to eat right or exercise regularly or meditate every day.

   * About anything!

2. **Start to think positively**

   * Focus on the thoughts and words you create, on how and what you are thinking and talking about.

   * Formulate sentences in a positive form.

   * Talk rather about pleasant things, such as success, love, happiness, perfect health as opposed to a lack of success or illnesses.

✳ Avoid criticism and humiliation. Instead of saying: *I'm fat and ugly!* say: *Every moment I become prettier and slimmer!*

✳ Even a rainy day can be beautiful if you let it. Instead of saying: *Gosh, raining again, it is awful!* say: *A lovely rainy day, ideal for exercise or meditation.*

✳ Protect yourself against criticism and negation.

· **First:** Limit watching the news and reading newspapers. They are full of negation that weakens you, whereas you need to strengthen yourself with positive thinking.

· **Second:** Choose those friends who support you and have similar interests.

· **Third:** Gently and lovingly teach positive thinking to your whole family.

· **Fourth:** Write down positive sentences in your journal and read them often. It is an excellent prevention, but also helps if you get into a negative mood.

· **Fifth:** If you find yourself in a group of people who are critical and pessimistic, then leave immediately and begin to clear your mind with positive phrases and visualizations of a funny situation. Take all the negative thoughts you absorbed there and throw them in the trash bin. Fill your mind with positive thoughts. If you can't leave the situation (for example, during a work meeting), then try to change the subject. Or, in the meantime, *"pick up"* a funny story from your own *"emergency archive"* and play it in your mind like a movie.

- **Sixth:** Meditate or visualize for at least 15 minutes a day. If you do not have time during the day, then try before bedtime or right after waking up.

- **Seventh:** Practice affirmations! The principle is simple. Repeat a positive phrase in the present tense aloud or silently (depending on your social situation), describing your success in relation to the problem or goal. For example, in the morning after waking up, I repeat the positive attitude: *Today is one of the most beautiful days of my life. Today miracles happen. Only goodness, love, health, happiness and abundance come into my life.* I also love the affirmation: *Good morning my body, I love you, I love your every single cell.* Other examples: *I love myself, I am on the right track, I am fit and healthy, I am beautiful.* Repeat the affirmation as often as possible. Aim for at least 100 times a day!

REMEMBER: EVEN IF YOU DO NOT BELIEVE THE AFFIRMATION AND IT STILL SEEMS LIKE A LIE, REPEAT IT! IMAGINE THAT THESE SENTENCES ARE

LIKE MAGNETS ATTRACTING EXACTLY WHAT YOU ARE AFFIRMING. EVERY CELL IN YOUR ENTIRE BODY WILL ATTUNE TO THE AFFIRMATION AND THE SENTENCE WILL GRADUALLY COME TRUE.

Wonderful! Now you know the rules for mastering your thoughts.

HOMEWORK:

Yes, exactly, please now take a highlighter and select two rules that attract you most and that you will apply to your life from this moment on. Also, make two copies of *the rules to master your thoughts* and hang one on the fridge and place the other on the nightstand.

Then, every second Monday take a highlighter and select one more rule. Write down this regular homework into your journal and calendar too!

Well done!

Don't think that I am done, that I have mastered all of my thoughts

No, I'm in the same learning process as you are now. I know very well that it's not easy to change your way of thinking overnight. Yes, I know. It's a matter of training, hard work and discipline. It's a lifelong process. You start with changing your thoughts about weight loss, and just as you improve that area, you find that you have room for improvement in your thoughts about relationships, and just as you improve your relationships, finances will come up. Every day I catch myself thinking about something negative. But the lovely part of it is that today I find my negative behaviour (thoughts) more quickly than yesterday and just as quickly fix it. It's like a sport. Training and practice, no matter if it is muscle or mind, improves my response and quality of life.

As I mentioned earlier in the book, I personally met the therapeutic method of positive thinking for the first time while reading the book: *You Can Heal Your Life,* by Louise Hay. I was 20 years old and devoured this book. I immediately started practising positive thinking and exercises described in that book and within a few days I saw amazing results. My life began to change. I am convinced of the positive outcome of affirmations and I really recommend reading the book *You Can Heal Your Life*, which I consider to be almost a bible for me. The author Louise Hay is a metaphysical lecturer and teacher with more than 50 million books sold worldwide. For more than 30 years, she has helped people throughout the world discover and implement the full potential of their own creative powers for personal growth and self-healing. She has appeared on The Oprah Winfrey Show and many other TV and radio programs both in the U.S. and abroad.

An important moment ...

Now you know 3 essential pillars on which my program and your lifestyle change is based. How do you feel?

Do you want more details? Well, don't rush, this is enough for starters. In my early days, I explained everything to my clients during their first consultation. But I don't do this anymore, because a large amount of information can be overwhelming and isn't a good way to start out. In my current practice, most of my clients leave my office with only three sheets of paper, with the roles of the three essential pillars of *Training of body and mind*, the three keys which together unlock the gate to success.

Of course clients ask questions and want to know more. But you know what? I tell them: *Go home and start doing your best. Concentrate your thoughts on it! Do not search for the why, do not doubt, do not cheat and do not change it, and come back after 2 weeks.* These 2 weeks are very important. During this time many changes at the body, mind and spirit level happen. And, most importantly, during these two weeks, many answers will come to the client naturally and automatically, without my help. And that's what I strive for in my coaching.

Well, you know, you too have to do the best you can, as soon as possible. I'm not saying go away and come back in 2 weeks! As I said, this is a different approach from my classic one-on-one coaching. As I promised, I will guide you step by step. Either way, without your actions, you will not do any progress, any change.

NOTE: AT THE END OF THE BOOK, IN THE CATEGORY OF BONUSES, YOU CAN FIND A SUMMARY OF THE RULES.

Notes:

_____

_____

_____

_____

_____

_____

_____

_____

_____

_____

_____

_____

_____

_____

Alright, in the following steps I am going to help you with one of your main goals, which is to **LOSE WEIGHT!**

I am sure you will find other very important rules that must be mastered to ensure your successful holistic lifestyle change.

Are you excited? Take a deep breath, we're going to take the sixth step!

Step 6

Calculate Your Optimum Body Weight

In this step you will find the approximate number that will help you get an idea of the recommended body weight corresponding to your height.

If you are a woman, then use the formula:

Height (cm) – 110 = approximate optimal TH = ...kg

If you are a man, then use the formula:

Height (cm) – 100 = approximate optimal TH = ...kg

I want (need) to lose ....kg

NOTE:

1 Pounds (lbs) is equal to 0.45359237 Kilograms (kg)

1 Kilograms (kg) is equal to 2.2 Pounds (lbs)

1 Centimeter (cm) is equal to 0.3937007874 Inches (″)

1 Inch (″) is equal to 2.54 Centimeters (cm)

Well done!

NOTE: THE PRIMARY AND AUTHORITATIVE INDICATOR OF PROGRESS IS NOT THE NUMBER ON PERSONAL WEIGHT, BUT THE BODY COMPOSITION AND BODY MEASUREMENTS!

REMEMBER: WEIGHING YOURSELF REGULARLY CAN HELP YOU DETERMINE WHETHER YOU ARE EATING THE AMOUNT OF CALORIES THAT YOUR BODY NEEDS. IF YOUR WEIGHT IS GOING UP, CUTTING BACK ON THE AMOUNT OF CALORIES YOU ARE EATING EACH DAY CAN HELP YOU LOSE WEIGHT. ALWAYS COMPARE YOUR WEIGHT HISTORY TO TRENDS IN YOUR CALORIE INTAKE AND PHYSICAL ACTIVITY!

Notes:

Step 7

Body Measurements

I find body measurements to be very helpful, simple and reliable indicators of progress.

Measure yourself without clothing. During measurement, keep your muscles relaxed. The metre should be lightly touching the skin.

I recommend that you measure seven points of the body:

1. Neck – Measure at half the height of the neck.

2. Arm – Measure the circumference of the mid upper arm when outstretched.

3. Chest – If you are a woman, measure the circumference of the chest just below the breasts. If you are a man, measure the circumference over the nipples.

4. Waist – Measure over the belly button.

5. Hips – Measure at the widest part of the hip joints.

6. Thigh – Measure at the first third of the femur from above.

7. Calf – Measure at the widest part.

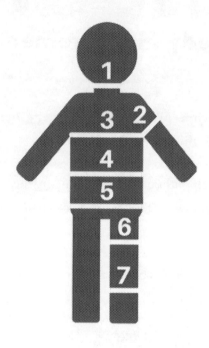

Body measurements

NOTE:

1 Centimeter (cm) is equal to 0.3937007874 Inches ('')

1 Inch ('') is equal to 2.54 Centimeters (cm)

Part / date						
1 (cm)						
2 (cm)						
3 (cm)						
4 (cm)						
5 (cm)						
6 (cm)						
7 (cm)						

Now, please take your journal, the pencil and the meter, and make the first measurement.

Done? You are doing great!

Notes:

_____

_____

_____

_____

_____

_____

_____

_____

_____

_____

_____

_____

_____

_____

Step 8

Deadline By Which You Will Lose Weight

The deadline must be set up realistically!

Please pay good attention to this step! Often in practice, I see that the deadline is just what people do not take seriously. Unfortunately, hope for success for those people then significantly drops.

How to determine the deadline:

In this case, we are talking about the goal of losing weight. So I will show you how to calculate the time you'll need for reducing as many kilograms as you have set up.

You have to think not only about how much time you will need to achieve this, but also take into consideration your current status, including the age, health, and current fitness level.

The rules to master your deadline:

1. Do not try to rush it. Do not try to postpone it.

2. You need to set up time for weight loss correctly and smartly because you want to maintain a healthy weight, not to gain all the kilos back! Is that right?

3. The goal is to adjust the body weight at the expense of body fat and build lean muscle mass at the same time.

4. Extremely quick weight loss always points to imbalance, poor nutrition, a wrong training plan, improper energy management, or lack of rest.

5. The first kilograms drop off fast and easy, but the final kilograms drop slow or sometimes not at all. That is why we have to assume low to moderate speed for your metabolism. In my one-to-one coaching, I can calculate the exact data.

6. Weight loss changes the body inside and outside.

7. Increased ratio of lean muscle mass changes the speed of metabolism and the amount of daily energy needed.

8. A person weighing more burns more energy compared to a person weighing less.

9. A person with a higher ratio of muscle burns more energy compared to a person with a lower ratio of muscle.

10. Muscles are heavier than fat.

11. At every stage of weight loss you must regularly check and reconsider the settings of the ratio between the energy supplied and burnt, which includes reconsidering the settings of the diet and training plan.

Calculation:

Weight loss that is considered to be healthy is approximately 0.5kg (1.1lb) per week.

I want to reduce the total of .... kg

Total reduced kg / 0.5 = number of weeks

Number of weeks / 4 = the number of months

Example:

I want to reduce the total of 20kg.

20kg / 0.5 = 40

40 / 4 = 10 months

Outcome: In 10 months my body weight will be 20kg less (while respecting the rules)

And now it is your turn:

.... kg / 0.5 = ... weeks

.... / 4 = ... months

Outcome:

In .... months my body weight will be .... kg less (while respecting the rules).

NOTE:

1 Pounds (lbs) is equal to 0.45359237 Kilograms (kg)

1 Kilograms (kg) is equal to 2.2 Pounds (lbs)

Yes, that is the approximate time needed to lose weight and meet your first goal (though each person is an individual with a different metabolism).

You might be thinking: "So much time spent on achieving only one goal!"

Remember that this is the very best step with which you can begin your new life! It's not about a number on a scale, but the journey to get there that will change your life.

I know that on your list there are several goals you want to achieve – weight loss, change in diet, regular exercise, free time, school, work, family, money. At this stage of your lifestyle change, we are working on weight loss. Therefore, right now do not worry about a new career, or improving financial income, or improving the relationship with a loved one. Stay fully focused on your weight loss goal. And do not be disappointed! Remember, everything is connected to everything. Working on one goal will simultaneously help with your other goals! You do not want to start to achieve all of them at once, because this will make you feel overwhelmed, under pressure, and stressed. In the beginning we agreed that you will change your lifestyle step by step, so let's do it! Trust the Universe and yourself that at the right place at the right time you will start working on the next goal that's right for you. With each day you're making progress.

However, we have not reached the top step yet. We still have to climb the two final and very important steps.

REMEMBER: STAY FOCUSED! STOP COMPLAINING! START THINKING POSITIVELY!

Two more steps to go! Ready?

OK, let's see what you need to learn in the ninth step.

Notes:

Step 9

Face Fear

Ok, so, here we are on an extremely important step. To win, to be satisfied and happy, you must learn to face fear.

Alright, there is one thing you need to prepare for in advance. On your way to a new lifestyle you are going to meet two characters called *FEAR* and *EGO*. They work hand in hand. Fear is actually a product of the Ego. They are going to make every effort to stop your success, because they know very well that your every other success makes you stronger, while they become weaker.

They will whisper lies to you like: It is not the right time to start losing weight yet, because Christmas is coming soon, your birthday is coming, you're going on vacation, you do not feel well, this is not the right program for you, you have a lot of work to do, child, school, mortgage, ... you need to save money (this last one is their favourite trick).

They'll also whisper: Do not exercise now, today, tomorrow, next week, because you are tired, you have to cook dinner, the children are at home, your husband is waiting.

NO, NO and once more NO! Nothing they say is true! The good news is it's nothing more than the voice of the Ego (fear) in your head. The bad news is if you do not learn to recognize fear and Ego, and how to get them under control, then they will always manipulate you.

Your true self is ready, the one who is constantly waiting to trip you up is Ego

Okay! I am going to tell you a story that explains a lot. A young man had a great business idea that would ensure his family's financial stability for the rest of their lives. But this realization would involve making some decisions and changes in his life. Let's watch the conversation between his true self and his Ego.

TRUE SELF: I have a great idea about how to make money and secure financial stability for my family for life. I will start a business. Yes, this is it!

EGO: Well, wait, wait, not so fast, consider the risks. Think twice. You just got married and need to furnish the apartment. You can't risk losing income. What if this new business venture fails? Furthermore, this was not your field of study! Therefore, it could cause complications. First, you have to expand your education!

Four years later ...

TRUE SELF: I have completed university and the apartment is furnished. Now I'm ready to start my business! I can finally begin. Great! I'm so happy!

EGO: Now? Not at all! What about your newborn baby? You cannot afford to leave work and risk losing money! Your wife needs help with the household, and if you start a business, you will not have the time. You have to wait a few years!

7 years later ...

TRUE SELF: Well, our son is now at school and my wife has gone back to work. It is the right time to start my business!

EGO: Now? You finally have some free time and money in the bank. Now you want to invest all your time and money in a new business? Well, maybe in a year or two. Do you want to risk your marriage?

About 11 years later ...

TRUE SELF: We have travelled around the world. We have saved money. Now I can really start my business!

EGO: Too late! Now it's too late! Haven't you noticed that your business plan was realized years ago by someone else? Oh yes, that person became very rich indeed!

Sad, isn't it? Unfortunately, this is the story of many people who haven't learned how to get their fear under control

Did you find any connection between the story of this man and your own life? I'm not just talking about the job and money but also about weight loss, about school, relationship, buying new clothes or cars. Have you ever been in a situation where you couldn't decide what to do until it was too late? For example, the car was sold or the dress went out of fashion. Are you the type of person who likes to postpone things?

Maybe you know people who talk about wanting to lose weight, but they never try. Or people who do try but quit after only a few days or weeks. Those people simply can't resist negative advice from the Ego, which has no other purpose other than to scare you, to tell you that you can't handle it, that everything will change in your life and that you will disappoint someone. Do not listen to it!

Your Ego lives because of your fear. Fear is a life-giving energy for the Ego. That is why it works tirelessly to convince you that you're inept, incompetent, unsuccessful, ill, ugly, uneducated, poor, and busy. The Ego says you can't do this and that, he/she is prettier, richer, more talented than you, it will hurt you.

What EGO is telling you is nonsense. It's just trying to scare you. The bigger your fear, the more powerful your Ego. Ego is also trying to control everyone who opts for a lifestyle change and weight loss. The Ego fears change, and doesn't want you to be your own boss. It does not want you to make decisions for yourself. It does not want you to wake up your true self, to feel good, love, be loved, happy, successful, wealthy and beautiful, slim and fit. It does not want to confess anything because it would mean its end. Ego will fight forever.

Rules to master the fear:

Keep this in mind. When fear, bad feelings and hesitations appear during your lifestyle change, remember the previous paragraph, and:

1. Immediately change your thoughts! Simply say: *No, I know it's you, Ego, and I will not let you control me! Here, now and forever, I am the boss!*

2. At that moment, do everything possible to tune in to joy and laughter.

3. Imagine a situation which will make you laugh – a scene of a comedy, a joke, whatever. Make a reservoir of funny situations in advance for such cases. It might help to imagine the Ego as a very tiny, naked, funny-looking character standing in front of you.

What is fear?

Fear is nothing huge, nothing supernatural. Fear is nothing more than an emotion, like anxiety, sadness, shame, frustration, joy or panic. Emotions are the notified feelings that can be pleasant (satisfaction) or unpleasant (disappointment). In other words, I could say that emotions are manifestations (reflections, mirroring) of thoughts on the body. Emotions cause us to feel excitement or calmness, tension or relaxation. Pleasant emotions occur in situations where we feel safe and sufficient. We have love, food, warmth, health, relationships, and work. Unpleasant emotions come in moments when we do not feel safe. When we do not have enough love or money, when relationships do not work, when we suffer from hunger, or when we are cold. We come back to the fact that everything is interrelated. You see how the level of thinking affects the level of the body? And the same applies in reverse order. Highly escalated emotions are manifested by changing the behaviour of an organism. Affecting the autonomic nervous system causes the mobilization (alarm) or demobilization (paralysis) of an organism through changes in metabolism, heart rate, breath, skin colour, facial expressions and gestures. Emotions can strengthen us (e.g. anger) or weaken us (e.g. fear).

REMEMBER: LIES (FEAR) ARE FOOD FOR THE EGO. THE MORE YOU FEED YOUR MIND WITH LIES, THE MORE YOU WILL BE AWAY FROM JOY AND HAPPINESS. LOVE IS FOOD FOR YOUR SOUL (TRUE SELF). THE MORE YOU FEED YOUR SOUL

WITH LOVING THOUGHTS AND DECISIONS, THE
FASTER YOU WILL BECOME HAPPY AND SATISFIED.
REMEMBER, LOVE CREATES MIRACLES!

HOMEWORK:

In the next two months focus on recognizing truth and lies.
Truth is represented by your true self = Love. Lies are represented
by your Ego = Fear. Every time you make decisions, slow
down and think and feel twice. Ask yourself which of the
arguments is true and which are only whispers of fear? Simply
throw out the products of fear in the bin and trust and follow
the products of love.

By practicing this technique as often as you can, your right
instinct, intuition will grow stronger. Intuition is a connection
to the Universe, God, energy, all being.

Trust me, everyone has the opportunity to learn how to
minimize the power of the Ego and maximize the power of
love (true self). You can do it too!

Tomorrow is a big day. Rest and sleep well. To reach the top
we still have one final step to climb.

Notes:

Step 10

Say Yes and Do Your Very Best

Your training is almost complete! It hasn't been so long since you opened this guide and started your journey. At this point you have done a lot of work. Wonderful job! I am so proud of you!

I would like to remind you once again that this guide teaches you fundamental rules of your weight loss and lifestyle change journey. Of course each of the rules (steps) could go into more detail but that is not the subject of this guide.

Looking back on what I have shown you so far, I think you may have heard some of the things before, but together we have organized everything into a clear plan of action.

Follow this plan without changes and breaks as best as you can for at least 8 weeks, ideally from now on. After 8 weeks, you will surely see and feel positive change to your body, emotions and thoughts. I am sure you will love your *new you* and will never want to go back to the *old you*. After some time has passed, life may show you a new path to take. And if your intuition says *YES*, then take it!

REMEMBER: YOU'RE A WONDERFUL HUMAN BEING AND THE ENTIRE UNIVERSE SUPPORTS YOU!

ALRIGHT, IT IS TIME!

FROM NOW AND FOREVER SAY: _YES!_, AND DO YOUR VERY BEST!

I WISH YOU SUCCESS AND THANK YOU VERY MUCH FOR OUR TIME TOGETHER.

Bonuses

Bonus 1

Summary of the Basic Rules of Training Body and Mind

Packet Version:

1. Keep your balance from now on!

2. Take care of your body, mind and spirit from now on!

3. Eat fresh and healthy food from now till forever!

4. Do regular strength and aerobic exercises from now on!

5. Do regular aerobic exercises from now on!

6. Stretch your body every day from now on!

7. Keep your daily journal from now on!

8. Meditate and visualize for at least 15 minutes a day from now on!

9. Do affirmations after waking up and during the day from now on!

10. Create positive thoughts from now till forever!

11. Follow your intuition from now on!

12. Face fear from now on!

13. Appreciate yourself from now on!

14. Do your very best from now on!

Bonus 2

Summary Of The 3 Essential Pillars

Nutrition:

* Follow the nutritional guidelines *YES & NO* in this book. In particular:

    - I restrict saturated fat to 20% of my total daily intake of fat.

    - I use/eat white sugar only in exceptional cases.

    - I use/eat white flour 1-3 times a week, no more.

    - I eat fresh vegetables or fruit in 2-5 servings per day.

    - I drink 2-3 litres of water per day.

    - My daily energy intake is divided into 3-5 smaller meals.

    - I eat smaller portions. I am using smaller plates for dinner. The size of the main meal fits into both palms aligned, size of snacks can fit into a palm.

- I do not eat carbs after 2pm.

- I eat dinner between 6-7pm.

- I do not eat after 7pm.

- I can eat one small meal regardless of the weight loss plan – once a week.

- I drink alcohol in moderation or only in exceptional cases.

Exercise:

* Do workout – strength (resistance) training – 3-4 x 45-60 minutes a week.

* Do aerobic exercise 45-60 minutes, 4-5 times a week. Keep your heart rate up to 60-70 percent of maximum.

Lifestyle:

* I restrict smoking by one third.

* I sleep 7-8 hours daily.

* I am eco-friendly. I recycle, eat organic, dress up and wash in organic as much as possible.

Thoughts:

* I support my self-love by affirming: *I love myself!*, in front of the mirror every day.

* I create positive thoughts.

Daily Journal:

* I measure and record my body measurements – twice per month.

* I record my body weight – every Monday morning before breakfast.

* I keep a journal about nutrition, exercise, thoughts, experience, goals.

REMEMBER: WRONG RULES OR NO RULES AT ALL ARE THE MOST COMMON CAUSES OF FAILURE.

Bonus 3

4-Week Beginner's Workout Program

Workout day A:

1. WARM-UP: 5-15 min. (elliptical trainer, bike ride, power walk and slow run)

2. STRETCHING: 5 min.

3. WORKOUT: 45 min.

Muscle group	Exercise	1,2 week	3,4 week
Back, shoulder	Supermans	2 x 12	3 x 12-15
Abs, Back, Hips	Bird-dog	2 x 20	3 x 20
Abs, Legs	Glute Bridge Single Leg	2 x 15	3 x 15
Abs	Crunches	2 x 20	3 x 15-20
Abs, Legs	Bicycle Crunches	2 x 12	3 x 12-15
Back, shoulder	Seated Lat Pulldown	2 x 12	3 x 12-15
Back, shoulder	Seated Machine Rows	2 x 12	3 x 12-15
Biceps	Seated Dumbbell Biceps Curl	2 x 12	3 x 12-15
Calves	Calf Raises	2 x 12	3 x 12-15

4. AEROBIC EXERCISE: 45-60 min. In moderate heart rate zone (60 to 70 percent of HRmax).

5. STRETCHING: 10-15 min.

Workout day B:

1. WARM-UP: 5-15 min. (elliptical trainer, bike ride, power walk and slow run)

2. STRETCHING: 5 min.

3. WORKOUT: 45 min.

Muscle group	Exercise	1,2 week	3,4 week
Back, chest	Cat-Cow	2 x 12	3 x 12-15
Abs, Legs	Glute Bridge	2 x 15	3 x 20
Abs	Sit-ups	2 x 20	3 x 20
Legs, abs	Reverse Crunches	2 x 15	3 x 15
Chest, arms	Dumbbell Incline Press	2 x 12	3 x 12-15
Chest, arms	Dumbbell Incline Chest fly	2 x 12	3 x 12-15
Triceps	Dumbbell Triceps Kickback	2 x 12	3 x 12-15
Legs	Seated Machine Leg Extension	2 x 12	3 x 12-15
Legs	Seated Machine Curls	2 x 12	3 x 12-15

Muscle group	Exercise	1,2 week	3,4 week
Shoulder	Seated One Arm Dumbbell Press	2 x 12	3 x 12-15

4. AEROBIC EXERCISE: 45-60 min. In moderate heart rate zone (60 to 70 percent of HRmax).

5. STRETCHING: 10-15 min.

Bonus 4

The Core Workout

1. WARM-UP: 5-15 min (elliptical trainer, bike ride, power walk and slow run)

2. STRETCHING: 5 min

3. WORKOUT: 45 min

Exercise	1,2 week	3,4 week
Supermans	3 x 30 sec.	3 x 60 sec.
Push Ups	3 x 30 sec.	3 x 60 sec.
Plank Leg Raises	3 x 30 sec.	3 x 60 sec.
Plank Arm Raises	3 x 30 sec.	3 x 60 sec.
Plank Twists	3 x 30 sec.	3 x 60 sec.
Up and Down Plank	3 x 30 sec.	3 x 60 sec.
Mountain Climbers	3 x 30 sec.	3 x 60 sec.
Glute Bridge Single Leg	3 x 30 sec.	3 x 60 sec.
Bicycle Crunches	3 x 30 sec.	3 x 60 sec.
Reverse Lunges	3 x 30 sec.	3 x 60 sec.
Side Kicks	3 x 30 sec.	3 x 60 sec.

4. AEROBIC EXERCISE: 45-60 min. In moderate heart rate zone (60 to 70 percent of HRmax).

5. STRETCHING: 10-15 min.

Bonus 5

Meal Tips

Breakfast:

* Oatmeal, fresh fruit, honey and cinnamon

* Quinoa, raisins, lemon, honey, nuts

* Slice of dark bread, low-fat cottage cheese, sliced cucumbers and radishes

* Low-fat yogurt, fresh fruit, honey, nuts

* Carrot salad with pineapple and lemon

Lunch:

* Whole wheat bread, butter, turkey ham, low-fat Swiss cheese, lettuce

* Whole wheat wrap, avocado, lettuce, tomato

* Rice pasta with tomato mushroom sauce

* Baked sweet potato with low-fat cream cheese, spring onions

* Seaweed salad and brown rice

Dinner:

* Grilled chicken breast, mixed green salad, yogurt dressing

* Mixed salad, hard-boiled egg, low-fat mozzarella

* Baked salmon with spinach

* Grilled turkey breast with grilled vegetables

* Tomato soup

Snack:

* One piece of apple or banana

* 2 slices of watermelon

* 3 pieces of plum

* 3 pieces of medium-sized carrots

* 1/2 cup of fat-free Greek yogurt

* 1/2 cup of apple chips

REMEMBER: KEEP IT SIMPLE!

Bonus 6

Weekly Menu Planner

Day Date	Break-fast	Snack	Lunch	Snack	Dinner
MON					
TUE					
WED					
THU					
FRY					
SAT					
SUN					

Bonus 7

Checklist (Step 1-4)

STEP		READ	STUDY	BEGIN
1	THE BALANCE			
2	RULES TO MASTER YOUR ORDER AND DISCIPLINE - JOURNAL			
	To buy your one nice journal			
	Track F-E-T-E-G every day			
	Track body weight every Monday			
	Track body measurement every second Monday			
3	RULES TO MASTER YOUR NUTRITION			
	Basic rules for healthy eating			
	Say YES to this food			
	Say NO to this food			
	Master your shopping list			
4	RULES TO MASTER YOUR EXERCISE			

	Strength training			
	Aerobic exercise			
	Stretching and relaxation			
	Make an appointment for a free fitness orientation in the gym			
	Master your fitness schedule			

Keep this list with you and when you complete each step/ homework, check it off. This will help you set the intention and purpose, keep the clarity, focus and willpower, for every single day as well as the entire program.

Bonus 8

Checklist (Step 5-10)

STEP		READ	STUDY	BEGIN
5	RULES TO MASTER YOUR THOUGHTS			
	Stop complaining			
	Start think positively			
6	CALCULATE YOUR OPTIMUM BODY WEIGHT			
7	BODY MEASUREMENTS			
8	SET THE DEADLINE BY WHICH YOU WILL LOSE WEIGHT			
	The rules to master your deadline			
	Calculation			
9	FACE FEAR			
	The rules to master the fear			
10	DO THE BEST YOU CAN			

Keep this list with you and when you complete each step/ homework, check it off. This will help you set the intention and purpose, keep the clarity, focus and willpower, for every single day as well as the entire program.

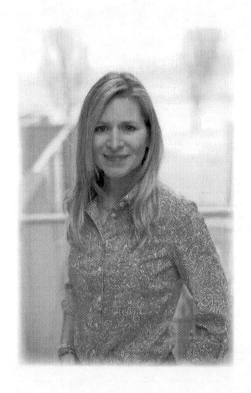

Daniela Gjurisic Lojkova

About the Author

Daniela Gjurisic Lojkova has been in private practice as a therapist, coach, healer, author, teacher and business consultant since 2002. With a passion to learn and teach about well-being, she has helped hundreds of people reach their wellness, fitness, health, personal and business goals. Her clients are people of all ages, from all over the world, including athletes, managers, celebrities, actors, politicians, businessmen, students, and coaches. Daniela is the author of a special wellness program called *Training of body and mind,* which teaches one of the possible ways to create wellness in body, mind, and spirit. To achieve and maintain better physical and mental health, fitness and weight loss.

Daniela is a co-founder of Alliance of Nutritionists of the Czech Republic, where she holds the position of vice-president.

She is registered with the leading educative company in nutrition Nutris® (Czech Republic) as a teacher of alternative nutritive methods. She is also a teacher of nutrition and wellness at the college in Prague, Czech Republic.

Daniela is author of the book called *Získejte rovnováhu těla, mysli, duše i ducha (Get balance of body, mind, soul and spirit)* published in Czech Republic, as well as of many professional articles, textbooks and lecture notes about wellness, fitness, personal training, nutrition, and coaching.

She has appeared at television, magazines and newspapers.

Daniela currently lives with her family in Canada in British Columbia.

EDUCATION: Bachelor's degree in sports and fitness; Diplomas: Manager wellness centre & day spa, Wellness activities instructor, Nutrition therapist, Personal trainer, Trainer of bodybuilding, Instructor of fitness, Massage therapist (Czech Republic). DotFit Fitness Professional, Reiki practitioner (Canada).

"My work in this world is teaching to create wellness in body, mind, and spirit."

Daniela Gjurisic Lojkova
www.danielagjurisic.com

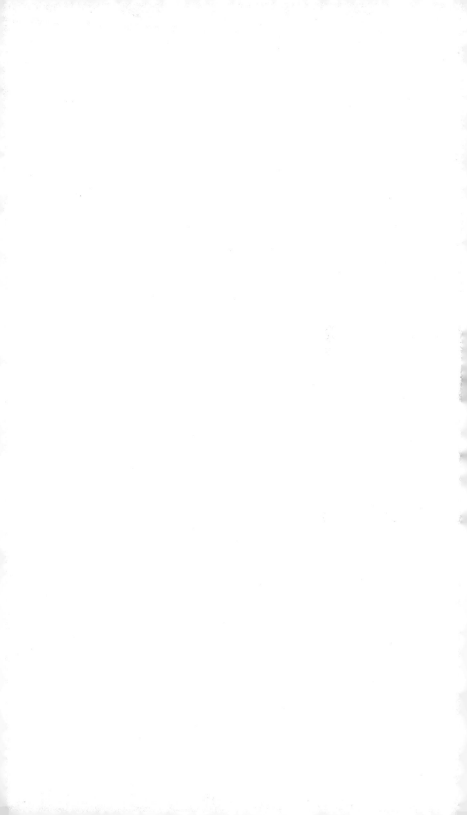

Printed in the United States
By Bookmasters